Dr. Earl Mindell's

What You Should Know About Beautiful Hair, Skin and Nails

Dr. Earl Mindell's

What You Should Know About Beautiful Hair, Skin and Nails

Earl L. Mindell, R.Ph., Ph.D.

with Virginia L. Hopkins

Keats Publishing, Inc.　　New Canaan, Connecticut

Dr. Earl Mindell's What You Should Know About Beautiful Hair, Skin and Nails is intended solely for informational and educational purposes, and not as medical advice. Please consult a medical or health professional if you have questions about your health.

Library of Congress Catloging-in-Publication Data
Mindell, Earl.
  [What you should know about beautiful hair, skin and nails]
  Dr. Earl Mindell's what you should know about beautiful hair, skin and nails / by Earl Mindell, with Virginia L. Hopkins.
    p.   cm.
  Includes bibliographical references and index.
  ISBN 0-87983-747-0
  1. Beauty, Personal. 2. Skin—Care and hygiene. 3. Hair—Care and hygiene. 4. Nails (Anatomy)—Care and hygiene. I. Hopkins, Virginia. II. Title.
RA778.M637   1996
646.7'2—dc20
                                                    96-6067
                                                    CIP

Printed in the United States of America

Keats Publishing, Inc.
27 Pine Street (Box 876)
New Canaan, Connecticut 069840-0876

99 98 97 96   6 5 4 3 2 1

CONTENTS

Contents

PART I:
Healthy, Beautiful Skin

CHAPTER 1

Getting Under Your Skin

Think of chapped lips, skinned knees, scalds and burns. The memories can make us wince. Think, too, though, of stroking, the warmth of sunlight and kissing. It is through our skin that we experience all these things, painful or pleasing. Skin, living and breathing between the worlds inside and outside our body, is messenger to them both. It's minus five and hailstones are pelting or that cat, soft and heavy on your lap, needs a claw trim: your skin can tell you both. When your nose turns blue with cold or you feel a stinging sensation, your skin is letting you know that your body reacts to these things. Our skin relays the changes, external or internal, and responses are triggered that restore the balance. We wrap a scarf around our face, rub on the lip balm, put the cat out and find an antiseptic lotion. This kind of basic functioning is easy to take for granted, and it is usually issues of health and appearance that bring skin more fully to our attention.

Have you ever worried about a friend looking pale and ragged with dark rims and bags beneath their eyes? Or perhaps you've comforted a feverish child, cooling their reddened cheeks and forehead? We instinctively recognize that skin condition is a sign of general state of health. Because skin is linked to so many bodily functions from blood circulation to excretion, it's no wonder that it can be a very clear indicator when things go wrong internally. Observing skin symptoms is sometimes the first step leading to treatment of major underlying conditions.

Of course, as a physical container and protector of flesh and blood, skin can have its own problems, too. Then the body has skin repaired: cuts are plugged, scabs formed and splinters and living invaders like bacteria are engulfed by extra blood flow, bombarding the site of injury with white blood cells and nutrients.

Technology advances, fashions change, but human fascination for skin and its appearance is constant. Ancient Britons used a blue dye from the woad plant as horrifying war paint; empresses are said to have bathed in asses' milk; European ladies and gentlemen of the 18th century powdered and rouged their faces; skin tattoos are popular the world over; plastic surgery is now big business; modern skin grafts are grown in lab dishes. This is not surprising, considering that looks are tied to emotions and sexual attraction. We go pale with shock and red with rage; we blush with embarrassment. Such indicators of emotional state combined with clues to health mean that skin becomes a physical factor in our relationships and also in the selection of a mate. In sex itself, skin plays a role, conveying and expressing the physical signals that lead to arousal. In fact, skin is easily the organ with which we are most intimately acquainted!

Our language ties qualities and values of skin to character traits and emotional reactions. We might refer to someone as "thick-" or "thin-skinned," or someone might get "under your skin." If something is of no consequence, you can say it's "no skin off my nose" or you might "scrape through" a serious situation and "save your skin." Recognition of the roles or importance of skin is built into our everyday lives. Often, however, our understanding and appreciation of its true work and nature are only "skin deep!"

Applying in-depth knowledge of skin functions can

lead not only to improving its condition and appearance, but also to overall well-being. Surface effects are resolved as deeper causes are addressed. In this way, healthy nutrition is a major factor in promoting healthy skin. A case of treatment from the inside producing real benefit on the outside. The scope and details of how this is achieved may be various, but, with skin, ultimately looking good usually means feeling good, too.

SKIN FACTS

- Dermatologists estimate that skin of an adult weighs about eight pounds and measures about twenty square feet when stretched out.
- The eyelids are covered by skin at its thinnest— only about $\frac{1}{25}$ of an inch.
- Skin can be around $\frac{1}{8}$ inch thick at sites like the soles of the feet.
- We shed around 40 pounds of skin over a lifetime.
- Men really are thicker-skinned than women!

YOUR SKIN IS YOUR LARGEST ORGAN

Nothing beats skin when it comes to waterproof protection for your entire body. This function alone, and the fact that it is a differentiated body part, would qualify skin as an organ. Yet its intricate structure exists to perform many tasks. Skin has two main layers, an outer band called the epidermis and an inner layer which is about four times thicker and known as the dermis.

The epidermis consists itself of three sub-layers. The topmost consists of scaly, dead cells, rich in protective keratin. Dead cells are shed constantly and are actually the major component of household dust. Newly generated cells move toward the surface, constantly replenished from the deepest layer of the epidermis called the basal layer. The basal layer also contains the pigment, or melanin, which gives skin its color.

New skin lies over the dermis, the skin's inner supportive layer. The dermis anchors blood vessels, sweat glands, sense receptor cells, hair follicles and oil-producing sebaceous glands. Sebaceous glands open out onto hair follicles, while sweat glands release their fluids through other holes in the skin known as pores. Beneath the dermis is a final layer called the subcutis, which is an insulating layer of fat.

COLLAGEN IS YOUR SKIN GLUE

Something has to bind all the structures of skin together, and this is done by a tough protein called collagen. Collagen is major component of connective tissue which is found wherever different tissues and body parts need to be bound. This protein is produced by cells in the connective tissue called fibroblasts. Collagen is formed in fibers which configure themselves in various ways, such as bundles ideal for the twisting and flexing of tendons joining muscle and bone. In skin, collagen fibers lie in a flat, crisscross position.

Collagen is the most abundant protein in the body. It is high in silicon, a mineral that forms long, complex molecules, suitable for parts of the body which need to be strong and flexible. Collagen works with fibers of another protein called elastin, which, as its name suggests, gives skin its elasticity. The two types of fiber together bring resilience and skin tone. Unfortunately, many people seem to produce less of these proteins as they get older, and factors such as sun and smoking contribute to their destruction. The result is aged skin, the target of numerous marketing campaigns for anti-aging cosmetics.

Some dermatologists recommend collagen injections for minimizing wrinkles and scars, and collagen-boosted lips have been acquired by some rich and/or famous women. Injected collagen is broken down by enzymes in about two years. Money spent on cosmetics with added collagen is also misguided since skin cannot absorb the protein. Nutritional support of our body's own collagen is a much more sound approach, and it can be delicious, too. Copper, found in dark, leafy vegetables, shellfish and whole grains, and vitamin C, abundant in fruits and vegetables, are both required for the production of collagen. Iron is needed, too, as found in organ meats, poultry, fish and parsley. In addition, research from the '80s shows that bioflavonoids, particularly PCOs, the powerful antioxidants, are very effective in stabilizing collagen structures.

SKIN IS YOUR BODY'S FIRST LINE OF DEFENSE

It's true, microorganisms are crawling all over us, new ones arriving every second! But thanks to our trusty skin, very few penetrate to levels where they can do harm. Germs from public contact are held off by healthy, intact skin. Bugs for illnesses such as colds and flu can only do their work if transferred to sites like our eyes and noses. Skin also filters the sun's rays and keeps out water and toxic substances. A more sophisticated barrier could not be invented.

Yet, besides its physical blocking qualities, skin forms an essential part of the immune system. In healthy people, the mildly acidic film of oil and sweat which coats the skin is itself slightly harmful to bacteria and fungus. Internally, many special cells called Langerhans cells are sprinkled throughout the skin.

The job of these cells is to catch viruses and bacteria and hand them over to white blood cells called T cells. Recent research shows Langerhans cells also interact with lymphatic fluid, or lymph, the clear watery fluid that transports white blood cells and other vital substances to blood and tissues.

New discoveries also show that a fascinating range of immune-related substances, such as growth factors, are produced by the cells lining the tiny blood vessels in the dermis. The interaction of all these agents has been observed to trigger complex signals and responses which provide protection against infections, abnormal tissue growth and external environmental toxins. As studies continue, it is seen that the cause of conditions like psoriasis may, in fact, lie in the skin's immune system turning against itself.

WHY SKIN IS YOUR NUMBER TWO DETOXIFIER

The skin has been called a second kidney as its millions of sweat glands excrete many substances that are toxic to the body. With vigorous exercise and high temperatures our sweat output increases from an average of about a pint a day to around eight quarts. It's no wonder saunas have become part of detoxification programs.

There are two types of sweat glands. Eccrine glands eliminate mostly water and excess mineral salts, including sodium chloride, which is why sweat tastes salty. These sweat glands work hardest with exercise, high temperatures or stress. Apocrine sweat glands are found in the genital region and armpits. They excrete nitrogen-containing wastes, as well as water and salts, through the pores of our skin. Apocrine glands are the ones to blame for body odor. The sweat from these glands creates body odor when mixed with bacteria and is produced at times of stress.

Poor diet can be a contributory factor in sweat glands becoming overproductive and clogged up. Sweat itself can become laden with material delicious to bacteria. Good nutrition helps the skin carry out its detoxification role and keeps down the levels of toxins it has to deal with.

SKIN, SOURCE OF NATURAL TONER AND CONDITIONER

You may have watched birds preening their feathers, spreading natural oil along the shafts and hairs to keep them waterproof and deter pests. When we brush our hair, we are doing the same thing! Our sebaceous glands produce a waterproof skin oil called sebum that is released along the hair shafts. The highest concentration of sebaceous glands is on the face, followed by the back, chest and shoulders, which is why these are the major sites for acne.

Sebum helps protect hair and keep it glossy while also preventing damage to skin from such factors as wind and dust. Sebum also lubricates the skin and prevents the loss of too much water. When skin retains the right amount of water, this helps it to stay supple. Most simple moisturizers work by supplementing the effect of sebum, sealing in the water content of skin, preventing its evaporation. Beware of too much washing or harsh cleansers, as these can strip away sebum, leaving the skin open to infection as well as dryness.

CHAPTER 2

Common Skin Problems

So many mechanisms are active in skin that it's easy to understand how their breakdown can result in numerous health conditions. Given the importance we attach to its appearance, it's also not hard to understand that skin problems often cause considerable distress, even when the associated discomfort is not great. The psychological relief gained from solving a skin problem is real and valid. The key is to not be pushed into harsh and desperate measures by the strong emotional drive to find solutions to conditions like acne. There are many gentle, natural remedies and supplements that help bring the chemistry of skin back into balance. Try these first and aim at a lifestyle without emotional roller coasters and low in stress—your skin reflects both!

SKIN TYPES

What skin type are you? Although you are born with a tendency to basic skin features, your answer may change throughout your life. Skin is in constant renewal, responding to internal and external influences. Aging may bring drying and thinning as skin functions slow down. An extreme climate and indoor heating can also dry out your skin. Dietary changes can bring vitamin and mineral deficiencies and sensitivities. Hormone changes, from puberty and pregnancy to menopause, can also affect skin condition. Normal skin is considered to be skin in balance—smooth, "plump," soft, and blemish-free. Fresh, even tone goes along with small to medium pores.

Sensitive skin is delicate, easily irritated by external agents. This skin type is typical of blondes with blue eyes, and of redheads. Prone to rashes and stinging, this sort of skin also burns easily in the sun.

Blemished skin is typical of teenagers and is characterized by an overproduction of oil. In later life, contributory factors can include diet, poor stress, poor elimination, intestinal flora out of balance, environmental conditions, allergies and cosmetics.

Fair-skinned people are prone to dry skin, which involves an underproduction of oil. If skin is thick, but pores are visible, water is called for. If skin is fine with barely visible pores, oil, and possibly water, is lacking. Dry skin can be rough and scaly, too, without any shine.

Oily skin is often thicker than other types, and has medium to large pores and a shiny appearance. A disadvantage is a tendency to clogged pores. Olive skin is typically quite oily, enjoying the benefits of youthful appearance and less vulnerability to environmental damage.

Combination skin can see a mixture of oily and dry characteristics on the face. Often the forehead, nose and chin areas can be greasy, while the cheeks and eyes are dry.

Skin care can change to suit as you add supplements, change your diet and increase sun and cold protection. Simple observation will tell you when to put away or take out the astringents or moisturizers. Keep in mind that skin condition is the result of many different processes. If you are not troubled by a specific skin problem, it's a good idea to use the supplements and dietary changes recommended generally for healthy, youthful looking skin. Bringing the functions of your skin back into balance will often result in a skin type closer to ideal.

ACNE

Acne is the most common skin problem. Psychologically, acne can be a real downer, often striking teenagers who are already going through emotional turmoil at puberty. Its main features are blackheads, whiteheads, pustules, inflamed red bumps called nodules or papules, and cysts under the skin surface. Scarring can occur when nodules break down surrounding tissue and as a result of damage done by tampering fingers. Acne breaks out mostly on the face, and also frequently on the back, chest and shoulders.

Acne sites, the most dense locations of sebaceous glands, give a clue to the nature of the condition which involves overproduction of sebum. Male sex hormones (androgens) such as testosterone stimulate the production of keratin and sebum. They also enlarge sebaceous glands. Levels of these hormones increase at puberty in both boys and girls, and are higher in males, which are the reasons why acne afflicts mainly teenagers and is most common in males.

Research shows that higher blood levels of testosterone do not always lead to more severe outbreaks. The underlying factor may instead be increased activity, seen in the skin of acne patients, of an enzyme that changes normal testosterone into a more powerful form. Bacterial balance also seems to be very important, with one study revealing increased blood levels of toxins absorbed from the intestines in people with bad acne. This results in more inflammation and tissue destruction because it disturbs the ratio of copper to zinc. Makeup, drugs and pollutants also aggravate acne.

Although the condition is complicated, a thorough

understanding actually opens more doorways to the treatment of acne. Nutrition, as always, is important. Although diet, including items like chocolate and fried food, is not a direct cause of acne, sticking to a diet low in fat, sugar, and refined carbohydrates such as cookies and cakes, will greatly ease the body's toxic load. Stick to unrefined whole foods and high levels of vitamin-rich vegetables and fruit. Avoid milk, too, as it is frequently high in hormones. Steer clear of iodine, as it can worsen acne. These measures boost the body's ability to fight the bacterial infection and repair skin tissue. Herbal remedies make effective topical treatments:

- Lavender or calendula—cleanse with rinses made from extracts of the essential oils of these plants.
- Tea tree oil—apply this essential oil to inflamed areas as this herb has proven as effective, without the side effects, as benzoyl peroxide.

For further recommendations on lotions, see the section "Soaps, Oils and Lotions for Beautiful Skin."

SUPPLEMENTS FOR ACNE:

- Beta-carotene—25,000 IU daily to help boost skin immune functions and increase skin tone.
- B-complex, stress formula—100 mg daily after eating. The stress formula is recommended as it includes extra amounts of B6 and B5. Vitamin B6 is particularly helpful to women with premenstrual worsening of acne as it plays a role in steroid hormone metabolism. A deficiency is itself associated with red and greasy skin. B5 boosts the adrenal glands and helps to lessen psychological stress.

- Vitamin C—1,000 to 3,000 mg daily, dose spread through the day, to boost the immune system.
- Vitamin E—(dry form) 400 IU, and selenium, 100 mcg, once a day. These are antioxidants working in partnership with zinc and vitamin A. A brazil nut daily is a good source of selenium.
- Zinc—15 mg daily between meals and apart from other supplements. Do not exceed 30 mg daily, as larger dose can depress the immune system. Low levels of zinc are typical for 13- and 14-year-old boys and are associated generally with the change of testosterone to its more active form.
- Black currant oil—1,000 to 2,000 mg daily as a supply of essential fatty acids (EFAs) hard to come by in food, but required for healthy skin function.
- L-cysteine—500 mg daily with vitamin C, half an hour before meals. This amino acid is a powerful detoxifier and immune system booster.
- Herbal infusions—red clover, dandelion and burdock root are all helpful. Red clover boosts the immune system, while dandelion is a good source of vitamin A, a known skin healer. Burdock and dandelion both cleanse tissue, working against acne-promoting microbes and the damage they do.

It can take up to 12 weeks to really bring acne under control, although some sufferers find relief comes quickly. Patience and consistency with a whole food diet and supplements bring a safer and more thorough remedy than resorting to long-term doses of antibiotics or treatment with vitamin A-based medicines which deplete the body and can lead to toxic side effects. Echinacea, taken internally, two weeks on and two weeks off, also helps fight infection. Persistence and a hands-off policy really pay with acne.

BODY ODOR

Body odor is produced when sweat from the apocrine sweat glands is broken down by bacteria. Armpits get particularly odoriferous because they, and the genital region, are where apocrine glands are found. Antiperspirants work by inhibiting the action of the glands. Most commercial products do this with harmful ingredients like aluminum salts or dyes, and are best avoided. America has seen at least eight common ingredients of deodorants and antiperspirants withdrawn in recent years, due to health risks. Deodorants usually mask or partly neutralize the offending smells.

Natural ways to reduce the amount of armpit bacteria include:

- Splashing with rubbing alcohol or the more gentle witch hazel.
- Herbal antiperspirants with antibacterial ingredients such as extract of green tea.

Supplements that help keep body odor under control include:

- Vitamin B complex—100 mg daily.
- Zinc—15 mg daily.
- Acidophilus—as per directions on container, to keep intestinal toxins down.
- Chlorophyll tablets or capsules—one, three times daily, can also be effective in controlling intestinal bacteria.

Cutting down on coffee is an additional measure that can help with body odor. If body odor is serious, chronic and does not resolve using the above suggestions combined with eating a good, whole-food diet, get a medical checkup as an underlying cause may indicate a more serious illness.

BURNS

Immediate immersion in ice water for five to ten minutes, with brief breaks, is the best treatment for burns. Head for the hospital in the case of severe burns. In minor cases, after ice water immersion, apply an ice pack intermittently over 24 hours to maintain a low temperature. The cold reduces blood flow, helps prevent leakage of fluid into injured tissues and lessens pain. Natural topical treatments for burns include:

- Vitamin E—apply the oil to help reduce scar formation.
- Aloe vera—apply directly from a cut split leaf. This herb is very soothing and cooling. It is also packed with skin-healing agents.
- Calendula tincture/ointment—apply to the burn for pain relief, antibacterial and antiseptic action.
- Raw honey—apply to the site. This burn therapy is being used in China and gaining much attention from Western doctors. Honey is antiseptic, soothing and healing.
- Ginger—mash the root, soak up juice with a cotton ball and apply to burn to relieve pain.

To speed the process of recovery from burns, the following supplements are useful:

- Beta-carotene—25,000 IU daily, for immune stimulation and tissue restoration.
- Vitamin B complex—100 mg daily. PABA (Para-aminobenzoic acid) in particular can reduce the pain of burns.
- Vitamin C with bioflavonoids—1,000 mg three

times daily will help new tissue growth and help prevent infection.

- Vitamin E—1,000 IU daily to promote healing and lessen scarring.
- Zinc, chelated or picolinate—50 mg daily, apart from other supplements, to stimulate wound healing.

Victims of serious burns may have a fortunate encounter with a paramedic team equipped with a new product developed in Australia called Water-Jel. A thick, slimy mixture of plant extracts, including eucalyptus oil, it fights infection and is applied in sterile dressings. It is also water-soluble, which helps in the cleaning of wounds. Its main use is in products like fire-protection blankets, since it resists temperatures of up to 2,000°F—a staggering example of the potential of natural substances.

CELLULITE

Cellulite is not a disease as such. It is a poor skin condition, unwanted due to its unsightly appearance. When skin affected by cellulite is pinched, it bulges and pits in what is known as the mattress phenomenon. Cellulite becomes a problem when the bulging and pitting are evident without a pinch test when the person is standing or even lying down.

More than 90 percent of cellulite is seen in women. In men, cellulite can be a sign of a deficiency in certain hormones. Female skin is structurally different: the fat cells underlying the skin are larger, more plentiful and arranged vertically rather than horizontally. The second layer of skin, the dermis, is thinner in females. These facts matter because cellulite is the result of excessive fat cells and a deterioration in the connective tissue made up of collagen and elastin, binding the layers of our skin together. How many fat cells we have is largely determined by what our mothers ate when we were in the womb!

One of the best ways to prevent cellulite is to keep only a thin layer of fat under our skins. Gentle weight reduction (gentle to avoid stressing connective tissue even more, which would worsen cellulite) and exercise can help lessen the condition. We can also do something about the state of the tissue. Lack of vitamins and minerals, aging and too much sun are all factors which cause connective tissue to weaken and the dermis to thin. Without strong boundaries in place, fat cells can move up into the dermis, causing the skin to deform. In fact, cellulite develops mostly on the parts of the body which show weight gain (increased fat) first, like thighs and buttocks.

To tackle cellulite, try the suggestions for improving varicose veins later in this section, watch the weight, and exercise. Massaging affected areas helps by stimulating blood circulation and smoothing disrupted skin structure. Work from the outside in toward the heart. Look for creams containing the plant bladderwrack for its soothing, softening and toning effects. Steer clear of fats and refined carbohydrates, and try these supplements, which, unlike many, have confirmed beneficial effects on cellulite:

- Cola vera cream—apply to affected areas for a caffeine-induced breakdown of fats that will help improve the skin structure.
- *Centella asiatica*—30 mg of the herbal extract three times a day will stimulate the growth of stable connective tissue and blood flow.
- Horse chestnut (*Aesculus hippocastanum*)—in two forms, aescin, 10 mg three times a day, and the bark of the root, 500 mg three times a day. These compounds are anti-inflammatory, build up the

strength of blood vessels in the skin and tone the blood.
- Glucosamine sulfate or Glucosamine/Mucopolysaccharide Complex, 1000 mg daily.

CUTS, SCRAPES AND OTHER WOUNDS

Always follow first-aid procedures when skin is damaged. Visit the emergency room if in any doubt. Once general health and safety is assured there are several herbal remedies for use on the spot, *externally only* unless otherwise specified:

- Aloe vera—apply gel directly from split leaf to cuts and scrapes. Aloe contains astringent and antiseptic agents among others necessary for wound healing. Its polysaccharides are thought to lie behind its ability to stimulate growth and repair of the outer layer of skin.
- Arnica tincture—apply directly or in a compress to *unbroken* skin in case of burns, and stings. Arnica is a natural pain reliever.
- Calendula tincture/ointment—bathe cuts and stings with tincture or apply the ointment for pain relief and faster healing through its antiseptic and antibacterial action.
- Echinacea tincture—apply tincture to insect bites and take one dropperful in water. This herb is an effective immune booster with a traditional use in America as a snakebite treatment. It also helps to prevent destruction of a natural barrier between harmful agents and healthy cells.
- Gotu kola tincture—apply to cuts to set in action a powerful combination of wound-healing compounds used successfully in many clinical studies, especially with surgical incisions. Gotu kola was even used in India and Indonesia to relieve leprosy.

If a wound is dry a cream or ointment is usually best, whereas a lotion or liquid is called for if the wound is oozing.

Once first aid has been completed, a healthy diet and supplements are a big help in healing skin. These three nutrients are key:

- Vitamin C with bioflavonoids—1,000 mg twice daily.
- Vitamin E (dry form)—400 IU daily.
- Zinc—15 mg daily.

These can be taken together, but apart from other supplements to avoid interfering with absorption of other nutrients. All three aid tissue repair. The vitamins work together and are both excellent antioxidants, helping to keep toxins at bay. Vitamin C is essential for tissue growth and repair as well as for fighting infections, and vitamin E and zinc are both wound healers. Recent studies have shown that another supplement, vitamin K, is useful in reducing bruising. It encourages leaky blood vessels to heal faster and is now available in cream form.

Once again, a good healthy diet is called for, as recognized by doctors of the American Academy of Cosmetic Surgery, who recently reported that even mild malnutrition can delay healing and increase scarring.

DRY SKIN

Sun, wind, soaps, cosmetics, medications—all causes of dry skin, right? True, but they all do damage in basically the same way. Our skin's natural lubricator and water conserver is sebum, the oil produced by sebaceous glands. External agents wear away this vital substance. In addition, our skin tends to produce less sebum with age. Sebum production declines in most people as early as their twenties. Less sebum means less moisture retention which leads to dry skin with its typical features such as stiffness, scaliness and flakiness. Some people have a genetic low-oil producing tendency, leading to dry skin, which often carries the advantage of fine texture and clear complexion. Naturally dry skin, however, tends to develop wrinkles and lines earlier than other skin types.

Skin in general will also sacrifice its need for water, as the major organs have first call on supplies. In this way, simple dehydration rather than lack of oil can also cause dry skin. Poor digestion of fats and oils or a simple lack of essential fatty acids will also contribute to dry skin, which can be tackled with dietary adjustments and supplements. Always seek medical attention for severe, chronic dry skin which does not respond to dietary and topical remedies. Occasionally, a more serious condition such as thyroid malfunction, is an underlying cause.

Dry Skin Prevention

Usually you can prevent dry skin, technically known as xerosis, by preserving your skin's natural oil with these simple steps:

- Don't bathe or wash too often, and avoid very hot water which can lead to the release of inflammatory substances in the skin, promoting dryness and soreness. Sponge-bathe odor-producing areas between less frequent baths or showers. Wash your face with a gentle cleanser at night, but only splash with cool water in the morning. This way, you encourage your skin's repair work, out of the sun and wind, at night.
- Avoid long soaks in hot baths. Hot water can irri-

tate skin, and we've all seen shriveled, prune-like skin from staying in the bath. This wrinkly effect is caused, ironically, by dehydration—the worst thing for dry skin.

- Do not scrub or rub. Scrubbing removes the skin's protective layers and rubbing can irritate dry skin. Avoid washcloths and always pat your skin dry.

- Always rinse well, especially on your face. It is important to remove all soapy residues, as these can leave a drying film over your skin.

- Avoid astringents and product ingredients which dehydrate the skin. Examples are talc and alcohol. There are now alcohol-free aftershave lotions for men.

- Use mild, herbal cleansers. Strong soaps and lotions, especially ones containing deodorants, actually strip sebum away. Lavender and chamomile, used for centuries in herbal baths, are soothing and antibacterial. Comfrey in particular helps skin to rejuvenate.

Moisturizers

As well as preserving sebum, you can support its action by applying moisturizers. It's important to find one that is allergen-free. If you are prone to allergies, be wary of lanolin, an oil from sheep's wool which is known to cause reactions in some people. Test moisturizer on a small portion of skin before using it generally.

The most common moisturizers are emollients—softening, soothing agents that usually contain fat. These work like sebum in that they seal in water already in the skin.

Other moisturizers contain humectants, substances that attract and hold water. Sodium hyaluronate (hyaluronic acid) is a humectant that can bind up to 1,000 times its own weight in water. Another good humectant ingredient to look out for is known as NAPCA. Our skin has its own moisturizers of this type, but slowing cellular processes mean these are frequently not produced in great enough number to prevent dryness.

Various claims are made for creams loaded with much-hyped ingredients from liposomes to amino acids. Ingredients like alpha-hydroxy acids (AHAs) are now being touted as valuable additions to moisturizers. Research published in *Cosmetics and Toiletries Magazine* shows that AHAs are not in fact particularly useful for skin hydration. What's more, many types of hydroxy acid (HA), not just the alpha kind, were found to be as effective. Look out, then for HAs and use them for their proven overall skin improvement, not specifically as a dry skin treatment.

The most effective ingredients are not necessarily the most expensive. So before you hit your pocketbook hard, try these proven natural remedies and remember, moisturizers work best when applied to damp skin.

Vitamin E, borage, black currant, flaxseed and evening primrose oils can work wonders as natural oils that moisturize and supply the skin with nutrients.

Egg-rich mayonnaise is a very good dry-skin moisturizer.

For really parched skin, mix up a moisturizing mask, using an egg yolk whisked with one teaspoon of canola or sesame oil and one tablespoon of honey. Ripe avocado also makes a beneficial mask. It can be mashed with egg yolk, or an equal amount of sour cream or ripe banana.

Dry Skin Nutrition and Supplements

Working from the inside to maintain your skin's natural protective coating is just as important as topical treatments. There is just no substitute for a nutritious whole-food diet, high in grains, fruit and vegetables. And keep hydrated! Aim at about eight glasses of unpolluted water a day, including herbal teas. In today's fast-paced, high-stress world, supplements like the following are also helpful in treating dry skin:

- B-complex—100 mg daily after any meal. Deficiencies of vitamins B1, B2, pantothenic acid or biotin can lead to dry skin problems and scaliness around the mouth and nose.
- Beta-carotene—25,000 IU daily, split between breakfast and after dinner. Your body makes vitamin A from beta-carotene without the risk of toxic overdoses. The benefits include soft, smooth and disease-free skin (a deficiency can itself produce dry, scaly skin).
- Vitamin C with bioflavonoids—1,000 mg two to three times daily after meals and at bedtime. This vitamin is always a good idea as it is required for tissue growth and repair.
- Vitamin E (dry form)—400 IU, one to two daily after meals. This supplement helps to replace cells on the skin's outer layer and works with vitamin C.
- Black currant oil—1,000 to 2,000 mg daily for essential fatty acids that promote good skin condition.
- Zinc—15 mg daily to aid skin tissue growth and repair, taken between meals and apart from other supplements. Zinc deficiency itself can cause dry skin with a rough, scaly appearance. Excessive sweating can result in a loss of as much as 3 mg a day of zinc.

- Glucosamine sulfate or Glucosamine/Mucopoly-saccharide Complex, 1000 mg daily

Black currant oil, beta-carotene and zinc are proba-bly the three most effective supplements for dry skin. It is also wise to consume plenty of omega-3 fatty acids by eating fatty fish. With good nutrition and cleansing underway, don't forget you still need to protect your skin from drying out as a result of the elements—wear those gloves and scarves in wind and cold, and sunscreen on bright days. Check out the section on winter sun for some more dry skin tips.

ITCHES, RASHES AND ALLERGIES

A rash is the name for the appearance of skin irrita-tion such as redness and blisters. Many rashes itch as the skin gives its lowest pain signal. The instinctive response of scratching increases blood flow to the region. This can be beneficial, although it also some-times spreads rashes. Some scientists believe scratching produces a stronger nerve signal which serves to drown out the original, more distracting itch. Rashes and itching are common symptoms of allergies. When the body responds to a substance which is normally harmless, skin cells release histamines which make fluid leak from tiny blood vessels into skin tissue. This is called an allergic reaction and in turn causes swell-ing, rashes and itching. Supplementation, topical treatments and dietary changes are used to bring the body's immune system back into balance or simply to calm symptoms like inflammation and itching.

Dermatitis, Eczema and Hives

Dermatitis is the term for an inflammation of the skin. It has many causes. Hives, inflamed weals or welts, are an allergic reaction, lasting a few hours or days, to things like sun, shellfish or berries. Hives are much less serious than eczema, which is a chronic inflammation of the skin named from the Greek for "to boil out." Itching, redness, small blisters, weeping and swelling are all features of eczema. Crustiness, scaliness and thickening follow. Eczema is the end result of many internal reactions to allergens. Children and young adults are most affected by eczema as a chronic condition, also known as atopic dermatitis, which is thought to be due to inherited hypersensitivities.

The results of a study in recent years at the Middlesex Hospital in London led researchers to conclude that excluding certain foods from the diet would alleviate moderate to severe cases of eczema in children. If eliminating cow's milk, eggs, tomatoes, artificial colors and food preservatives doesn't do the trick, look for another frequently eaten food to cross off.

Another study of atopic dermatitis at the University of California at San Francisco showed that sufferers can be helped by taking extra vitamin C. Patients taking the supplement for three months saw the number and severity of symptoms, as well as infections, reduced. If you have eczema, be sure to eat those fruits and vegetables!

Sensitivities—From Plants to Antiperspirants

Eczema-like rashes are seen in cases of poison ivy, poison oak and reactions to other plants as well as to things like solvents, nickel, lanolin, antiperspirants, and soaps, which can all be allergens. These kinds of reactions are known as contact dermatitis. They are caused by sensitivities and are not true allergies. Stress, heat, soaps, scratching and rubbing can worsen rashes. Diet, especially milk, can play a role, particularly with children. Always avoid an allergen once it is identified.

Plant oils, in particular, are very long-lasting. Contact with plant oils brushed off onto clothing, tools, and so on will cause further reactions, so be sure to thoroughly wash any items possibly contaminated. Nickel jewelry can be varnished with clear nail polish, or the skin under watches or bracelets can be dusted with talc to lessen contact. Always ensure that ear piercing is done with stainless steel needles.

Bringing Relief from Itches, Rashes and Allergies

When it comes to treatment of severe rashes, steroid creams and oral antihistamines are often administered and do bring relief. However, they do not address underlying causes and do create side effects. They are for short-term use only. Herbal treatments, supplements and dietary adjustments are much safer and gentler. For topical relief try these:

- Zinc ointment (non-oily)—apply to the skin three times daily.
- Aloe vera—apply gel from leaf to skin to cool, soothe and aid healing.
- Herbal ointment—containing licorice or German chamomile for their anti-inflammatory, cortisone-like actions.
- Herbal bath—chamomile, lavender and even oatmeal are all soothing and healing.
- Mugwort plant—for poison oak prevention and relief: After washing off the affected area (if possible), rub leaves on skin as soon as possible after contact. Steep fresh leaves in just boiled water for ten to fifteen minutes. While the remedy is brewing, take a shower, followed by a ten-minute soak in a bath containing the mugwort infusion. Avoid contacting clothes as much as possible while re-

moving them and place them directly where they can be washed separately from other items.

For internal support, the following supplements can be taken:

- Vitamin B complex—stress combination, with breakfast and dinner.
- Pantothenic acid (vitamin B5)—500 mg one to two times daily to support the body's anti-inflammatory actions launched by the adrenal glands.
- Vitamin C—500 mg four times a day as a natural antihistamine and also because histamines destroy vitamin C.

For severe rashes and eczema in particular, the above and following supplements are useful:

- Beta-carotene—25,000 IU daily, for up to a month, reducing to 15,000 IU for maintenance, for skin repair.
- Bioflavonoids—500 mg daily as antioxidant support.
- Vitamin E (dry form)—400 IU daily as a skin repairer and anti-inflammatory.
- Zinc—15 mg daily, for tissue repair.
- Evening primrose oil—1,000 to 3,000 mg daily.
- Herbal infusions—yellow dock, burdock, red clover, figwort, fumitory, heartsease, echinacea (purple coneflower) all help to nourish and cool the blood and skin. Borage and licorice aid the adrenal glands.

Oil of evening primrose is recommended for eczema sufferers, as they appear to be low on essential fatty acids which are needed for the body's antiinflammatory mechanisms. Omega-3 oils also supply fatty acids, and a diet rich in foods like mackerel, herring and salmon, nuts and seeds is a good idea for anyone prone to rashes, allergies and itching.

LIVER SPOTS

Often confused with age spots, liver spots are yellow, brown or black flat freckle-like marks on the skin, most prevalent in elderly people although they also frequently appear around age 40. Age spots look similar, but have irregular surfaces and look "pasted on." They are thickened areas of skin involving sebaceous glands which means they arise on the face, neck, chest or upper back. Age spots often itch and are usually harmless, though they are removed by doctors since they can be precancerous.

A true liver spot is called an *actinic lentigo*, from the Latin for "ray" and "lentil" In other words, a spot, small and round like a lentil, caused by too much exposure to the sun's rays. They can actually be up to an inch in diameter and do sometimes resemble liver in color and shape. Liver spots are seen mostly on the face or the back of the hands. They involve irregularities of the skin's pigment, melanin. The coloration of a liver spot goes deeper than a freckle.

Although liver spots are not usually a sign of disease, seek medical advice if any begin to change in any way. Research is ongoing into drugs which may lighten or remove liver spots, as people feel they are unsightly. You might have heard of Retin-A or Tretinoin, names for retinoic acid. This drug is a vitamin A derivative much hyped in the '80s. In fact, although there are positive results in studies with creams containing this drug, improvement tends to be modest and brings the risks of an increased tendency to sunburn, dryness, acne flare-ups and irritated skin.

If you find liver spots hard to live with, remember they are a useful warning of too much sun. Eat a carrot a day or take a beta-carotene supplement to help your body produce its own vitamin A and follow the advice for keeping your skin healthy in the sun. Avoiding excessive sun exposure is the best treatment of all, according to the American Academy of Dermatology.

VARICOSE VEINS

When the delicate walls of veins are damaged, the veins widen and the valves inside them become faulty. Veins then become varicose, that is, twisted as well as further widened. As well as being unsightly when they show through the skin, varicose veins can be accompanied by fatigue, aching and a feeling of heaviness. They are seen mostly on the legs, affecting almost half of middle-aged adults and four times more women than men. Pregnancy is a major cause of varicose veins, due to increased pressure in the veins of the legs. The condition is serious when it affects veins deep in the leg, bringing risks of clotting, heart attacks and strokes.

Genetic weakness of valves is thought to contribute to varicose veins, but theories about causative factors exist concerning ways that walls of veins become weakened. Keeping the skin conditioned is important, since skin helps to support and anchor many veins. Take note that the condition is rare in areas of the world where whole-food, high-fiber diets are the norm. Use the effective herbal remedies proven to relieve cellulite as these also work well on varicose veins. The steps below will help you keep your venous system healthy:

- Get plenty of exercise.
- Eat lots of fruit (especially berries), fiber, garlic, ginger, onions and cayenne—all good food for the circulatory system.
- A good preventive measure for varicose veins is to keep weight down.

Recommended supplements include:

- Vitamin E (dry form)—400 to 800 IU daily.
- RNA/DNA—100 mg daily.
- Grapeseed extract—150 to 300 mg daily as a rich source of PCOs which are powerful antioxidants that help to strengthen blood vessels.
- Zinc—15 to 30 mg daily to help keep tissues strong.

CHAPTER 3

Healthy Skin By the Season

HEALTHY WINTER SKIN

Winter skin problems are not caused by lack of sunlight. In fact, this time of year can be a good opportunity for your skin to rest and recover from long doses of high ultraviolet summer light. So please don't bask under tanning lamps as a solution to winter skin problems! They will definitely do more harm than good. The most common unwanted winter skin condition, especially for older people, is dryness. Read the section on dry skin for some general hints on care and prevention of this condition. Winter brings particular challenges though, which are worth attention.

Winter, Vitamin C and Collagen

The immune system benefits of vitamin C make it a useful supplement in winter. It's a wise measure for your skin, too, since vitamin C is essential for the production of collagen. Researchers looking not at skin but at vascular disease, have actually found a seasonal connection for vitamin C. Their year-long study, published in the *Scottish Medical Journal*, found that levels of vitamin C in the white blood cells of subjects dropped in winter. Boost your skin's collagen with a generous supply of vitamin C in your winter diet. Eat plenty of oranges, and take a vitamin C supplement of 500 mg at least three times a day.

Winter, Antibiotics and Biotin

Fall and winter typically bring bouts of illness all too often treated with antibiotics. Antibiotics destroy B vitamins, including biotin, and hamper the ability of intestinal flora to make this essential nutrient. This makes antibiotics the most likely cause of a biotin deficiency, and one of its signs is dry skin. As always, then, be very certain of the need for antibiotics before you take them. If antibiotics are necessary, a vitamin B complex supplement is too, for general health as well as dry skin. Take a B complex, because they work with each other in balanced partnership. Good general insurance against a biotin deficiency is to eat foods like eggs, peas, nuts, molasses and whole-grain cereals. Also keep intestinal flora in good shape with acidophilus supplements to aid synthesis of biotin in the gut.

Winter and Humidity

A snap of cold winter air can be bracing and refreshing, but it is also drying. At the same time, the indoor comfort of central heating only increases the wrinkling, shriveling effect, as dry air and heat both promote the loss of water from the skin. Chapped skin, as seen, for instance, in cracked and peeling lips, is a telltale sign of winter dryness. Applying lip balm and moisturizers helps prevent symptoms, and measures previously suggested for cuts and scrapes make effective remedies for chapped skin. To counter skin dehydration, take the steps recommended for dry skin, including moisturizers, supplements, healthy diet and protective clothing.

Avoid extremes—keeping your house at 85 °F and going out in your slippers and housecoat when it's below freezing are both ways to promote dry skin! In some homes, relative humidity is similar to that of

IN A NUTSHELL: 10 TIPS FOR HEALTHY WINTER SKIN

1) Drink plenty of clean water, about six to eight glasses a day. Dehydration is hard on the entire body, but it shows first on your skin. Your body is more than two-thirds water and your skin is the largest organ of your body. Skin is constantly handling incoming bacteria and releasing toxins through perspiration. Giving it plenty of water helps it do the job of housecleaning. At the cellular level, plenty of water is essential for the fluid balance and the exchange of waste material.

2) If you're breathing very dry air, get a humidifier. Indoor heating systems tend to dry the air, which dries your mucous membranes, making them more susceptible to infection. A humidifier is good for your sinuses, lungs and for cold prevention. You should have one in the room you spend the most time in during the day (which may mean taking one to the office), and one in the bedroom.

3) Use moisturizing lotions with vegetable oils—avoid mineral oils which clog pores. Try the new lotions containing NAPCA, a humectant which helps the skin retain moisture.

deserts! The Consumer Product Safety Commission recommends an air moisture level of 30 to 50 percent. This is usually comfortable, and plants and furniture will benefit, too. Keep temperatures reasonable, mist-water plants, and if you do use a humidifier, keep it scrupulously clean.

Winter Skin, Light and Vitamin D

Typically, only a small amount of vitamin D comes from dietary sources, including liver, egg yolks, fresh milk and fatty fish. More is produced when a particular kind of cholesterol is converted by the action of ultraviolet rays in sunlight on the skin. In a study on

4) For rough, chapped spots, open a vitamin E capsule and rub directly on the area.

5) Get plenty of omega-3 fatty acids by eating fish such as salmon, mackerel, cod, halibut, albacore tuna, sardines and herring at least twice a week, or taking supplements of borage oil, black currant oil, or evening primrose oil. These beneficial oils work at the cell level to keep skin smooth and supple.

6) Try lecithin to keep skin cells flexible. You can sprinkle lecithin granules on cereals or salads or eat them straight.

7) And while we're on the subject of oils, avoid the hydrogenated oils and the trans-fatty acids found in refined vegetable oils and margarine (not including canola oil or olive oil) which contain toxic oxidative molecules that cause aging and compete with the beneficial omega-3 fatty acids for cell receptors.

8) Wear gloves whenever it's cold out. Cold, dry air pulls moisture out of skin, aging it faster.

9) Drink alcohol in moderation. It's a vitamin robber and skin ager.

10) White snow is a highly reflective surface for bright sunlight. If you're spending more than 30 minutes outside in the snow, be sure to wear a sunblock with an SPF of 15 and sunglasses.

vitamin D, just 200 IU daily of vitamin D was shown to be enough to promote anticancer acitivity in the blood. Young children on a vegetarian diet might need a vitamin D supplement, especially in winter. Usually, however, deficiency of vitamin D tends to be a problem only for those who don't get out or who live in far northern countries.

HEALTHY SUMMER SKIN

Summer. We welcome its warmth and brightness on our skin. Increasingly, though, we set limits on that welcome, recognizing sunlight as wonderful in small doses and harmful in large ones. Now that pollution has thinned the ozone layer, caution is even more our summer skin watchword.

Keeping Your Skin Healthy in the Sun

The most important step you can take to preserve the health of your skin is to protect it from damage by sunlight. The American Academy of Dermatology is convinced by research evidence that exposure to the sun, rather than aging, is what causes most wrinkles. Sunburn afflicts millions of people every year, and skin cancer is on the rise. All this harm is caused by invisible rays known as ultraviolet (UV) light. Some researchers also believe that infrared or heat rays may increase the damage done by UV light.

The shorter, less numerous UV rays are called UVB, while UVA rays are greater in number and less intense. UVB attacks the top layer of skin, and is the most important cause of skin aging, skin cancer and sunburn. UVA is now thought also to be a major factor in skin aging, skin cancer and immune damage. It does not cause sunburn, but penetrates the deepest layer of skin, causing harm to elastin and collagen and damaging surface blood vessels. In this way, it destroys protective antibodies in the skin, causes older-looking, wrinkled skin and initiates disease. Sunscreeens that block only UVB may lead to users staying far too long in the sun without the burn caused by UVB, but with the initially invisible harm done by UVA.

UV light is most intense at the hottest times of the day in summer months, UVA in particular increasing in intensity by about 100 times. Levels of UVA remain potentially dangerous all year even in colder months. Beware of water, too. UV rays penetrate water to a depth of at least three feet, and water's reflective power amplifies sunlight. Snow also reflects UV rays and glass is no barrier to them. In addition, fog, smog and clouds do not provide an adequate block to the sun's harmful UV rays. As much as 80 percent of UV light still penetrates on overcast days. These are the reasons many skin experts now advocate the use of sun protection all year.

Medications and Other Products Can Increase Sun Sensitivity

It's not well known, but harm caused by sunlight can be magnified in some people taking medications such as antibiotics, antihistamines, diuretics, oral contraceptives and tranquilizers. Beware of aftershave products, colognes, cosmetics and soaps as well as products containing sulphur, benzoyl peroxide, salicylic acid, or resorcinol. After just a few minutes in the sun these can sometimes trigger a burn-like rash.

Unfortunately, sunscreens can also act as allergens. PABA, for instance, is a recent sunscreen ingredient to which some people are sensitive. If you develop a rash or burn when using a sunscreen, change it immediately.

Some Facts About Skin Cancer

Skin cancers usually start as tumors in the outer layer of skin which can grow and spread beyond their point of origin. The tumors are formed from cells that have been triggered into abnormal, out-of-control growth. UV light is the usual trigger for skin cancer. There is little doubt that more of the sun's damaging ultraviolet rays are reaching us as pollution has thinned Earth's protective ozone layer. Skin cancer incidence has been rising, particularly in countries like Australia where the ozone layer is thinnest.

Although sun exposure is responsible for some skin cancer, an individual's risk also depends on skin color, sex, and location. For example, skin cancer is more common in men, presumably because more men work outside. Rates of malignancies of the lips and face are lower in women probably due to protection from lipstick and other makeup. Skin cancer in Minnesota is 5.7 times less common than in Texas. This is because rates of skin cancer double every four degrees closer to the equator. Living at high altitude also increases risk, since it increases exposure to high-density ultraviolet light, which can trigger skin cancer.

However, cure rates for skin cancer are high. Different types of skin cancer are named after the type of skin cells they affect. About 95 percent of skin cancers are basal and squamous forms which have a matching cure rate of over 95 percent. Squamous cancers are potentially more dangerous, since they are more likely to spread. The most serious form of skin cancer, malignant melanoma, is responsible for 75 percent of all skin cancer deaths. Note, though, that only about 5 percent of skin cancers are this type and it has a cure rate of 90 percent when caught in its early stages.

While cure rates may be reassuring, they don't mean that skin cancer rates are not alarming—they are a definite indication of the increasing need to protect our skin from sunlight. Prevention of skin cancer is a matter of taking sun in low doses. Chronic overexposure does the really serious damage. However, avoid even the occasional burn, as just three blistering burns in your teenage years, for example, can increase the risk of skin cancer even five to twenty years after the original exposure.

Some Warning Signs of Skin Cancer

Older people should always check skin all over at least once a year. Those who have had skin cancer should check every six months. Everyone needs to keep an eye on any skin abnormalities, watching for new ones and changes in old ones. There are five basic warning signs for the most common type of skin cancer:

- An open sore that will not heal for three weeks or more.
- A persistent painful or itchy reddened area which may crust over from time to time.
- A smooth growth with a raised edge.
- A pearly or semi-transparent mole-like nodule that can be red, white, pink, brown or black.
- A white or yellow scar-like area.

The earlier skin cancer is caught, the better the chance of a cure, so be sure to visit a doctor if you develop any of the above symptoms.

No Such Thing as a "Safe" Tan

Dark, dusty, cramped surroundings became the norm for millions of workers with the coming of the industrial revolution in Europe. The wealthy were not confined to factories and could take vacations. A tan was no longer the mark of a farm worker or peasant. Instead it became a mark of affluence and fashion. This reversed the glamorous associations made until then with milky-white skin. Working conditions have long since improved, but the psychology of tanning has stuck, despite the ever-increasing evidence that sun is the number one cause of skin damage. A tan does signify the body's own protection against the sun's rays, but it is simply not enough, particularly in the face of environmental degradation.

Melanocytes are skin cells which produce the pigment, melanin, that colors our hair, eyes and skin. Uneven melanin distribution is the cause of freckles and liver spots. Sunlight stimulates melanin production which leads to tanning. The permanently high levels of melanin enjoyed by people with dark skin is the reason they suffer from much lower rates of skin cancer—whites contract 27 times more skin cancer than blacks.

Immunity and Sun

A report in *Cancer Weekly* covers research from the University of Texas and the Oregon State University on the effects of sun on the immune system. Studies with mice showed a 100 percent increase in tumor incidence in animals subjected to chronic UV exposure. One of the conclusions of the research was that sunlight can knock out some of the body's immune response to cancer. This, combined with UV damage to cell DNA, could allow cancer to form. Research of this kind leads many dermatologists to argue that a tan is actually a sign of skin damage and a warning to lessen exposure to sun.

It also supports observations about skin cancer and the state of the atmosphere. As the ozone layer has thinned, the age of patients with skin cancer has dropped as those seeking treatment are often in their late twenties and early thirties rather than their late forties and fifties. This has been a finding at the Department of Immunology of the M.D. Anderson Cancer Center at the University of Texas. The chairman of this department also warns that thinning ozone will lead to exposure to more intense UV, and further weakening of the body's immune system. In turn, this could result in more people becoming susceptible to different diseases and allergies. Sunscreen with both UVB and UVA blockers is highly recommended to help prevent immune impairment. Keep taking your antioxidants, too, for it is thought that sunlight stimulates the production of harmful free radicals which are neutralized or scavenged by antioxidants.

Sun Protection

Your first priority in sun protection are physical and chemical barriers to UV light. If you have children, remember that protection should begin early in life, not simply to avoid the pain of sunburn, but also because childhood burns can set the scene for trouble in later life. Follow these suggestions to increase your sun protection:

- Sun avoidance—I don't want you to avoid the sun altogether. For optimal health, you need some direct sunlight on your skin on a regular basis. Just make those sessions short and during times of day when the sun is less intense.
- If you're going to be out in the sun for a long time, wear a long-sleeved shirt and long pants.
- Hat and sunglasses—a large brim or nap is a good shield for shoulders and neck. Sunglasses with UV protective lenses are the only really effective choice, and worth the extra expense. But again, don't go to extremes. Your eyes need some direct exposure to sunlight. Don't wear your shades 100 percent of the time.
- Avoid sun-sensitizing substances, as mentioned earlier.
- Sunscreen—to be used routinely, even in shade, with a sun protection factor (SPF) of at least 15.

I want you to use a good, natural sunscreen, as some of the ingredients in cheap sunscreens can actually harm the skin with long-term use. It is essential to buy a sunscreen which blocks both UVA and UVB. Good sunscreens not only absorb both types of UV rays, they supply the skin with nutrients and help it to repair. Look for sunblocks containing free radical fighters and healers like zinc and vitamins C, A and E. A report in *Medical World News* focused on studies of the sunscreen effects of topical vitamin C. Studies show that this vitamin has sunscreening properties which lasted three days in animals, even after scrubbing. Vitamin C also seems able to provide protection without blocking the skin's ability to make vitamin D, and may also stimulate the production of melanin. While a safe, workable form of vitamin C as a sunscreen has not yet been developed, sunscreens enriched with this nutrient are a worthwhile investment.

Supplements for Sun

Taking supplements will not protect you from the sun's damaging rays. Only clothing and sunscreen can do that. What supplements can do is strengthen your skin's immune response and its tissue growth and repair mechanisms. There is no substitute for avoiding sun exposure, but a healthy diet and supplements, together with sunscreens and good sun gear, will help keep your skin healthy outdoors. All the following nutrients are needed for tissue repair, healing and reduction of scar tissue:

- Beta-carotene—10,000 IU daily.
- Vitamin C with bioflavonoids—2,000 mg daily.
- Vitamin E (dry form)—400 IU daily.
- Zinc—15 mg daily at night.

- Selenium—a Brazil nut daily is a useful source of this vitamin, or take a 200 mcg supplement.
- B-complex—100 mg daily, particularly for pyridoxine, vitamin B6, which has been shown in studies on mice to increase resistance to melanoma tumors and, in cream form, to reverse the development of human malignant melanoma nodules.

CHAPTER 4

How to Keep Your Skin Looking Young

When it comes to keeping young-looking skin, sorry, but moisturizers alone just won't do it. Moisturizing does plump up dehydrated skin and this does make wrinkles harder to see. However, simple rehydration doesn't address other major biological processes involved in aging skin. As time passes, it is usual for cell growth and glands to slow down. Typically, this will leave skin dryer, but also with less immune protection and weakened physical structure. Signs of aging, such as wrinkles, often start to show from around age 30. This all sounds drastic, but a healthy lifestyle with a whole food, high-fiber diet, lots of exercise and appropriate supplements really do promote youthful-looking skin. However, the slowing of cellular and glandular processes over time is not the most important factor in creating aged skin. Studies show that the sun is in fact the number one cause of an aged appearance, some experts reckoning that it lies behind 90 percent of all wrinkles.

Experts say age-caused wrinkles are fairly subtle, while those caused by UV radiation can be deep and extensive, as abnormal protein growth builds up, often lending a yellowish tinge to skin. The way the sun's light produces wrinkles and generally damages skin is known as photoaging and it can accelerate true aging effects by as much as twenty years! Read on for tips about natural aging, but also take sun seriously and less often, using the suggestions for healthy summer skin to keep those sags and wrinkles at bay.

Signs of Aging Skin

Thinning, fragility, wrinkles and loss of elasticity are all signs of aging skin. The binding between skin layers and nerve fibers, and circulation can all deteriorate with time. The outer layer of skin can become loosely attached and so more easily scraped and torn. Weakened blood vessels mean a greater tendency to bruise. Thinning of skin layers creates less insulation, bringing increased risk of hypothermia. Overall, less internal quality leads to less resistance to external factors, so older people tend to be prone to skin conditions in general, especially those related to long-term exposure to sun. Malnutrition is frequently seen in the elderly, and is often a factor which worsens late developing skin conditions. Begin those good nutrition habits now!

Antioxidants and Aging Skin

Many of the downhill changes associated with aging skin feature the destruction of cell membranes. Behind this biological damage are two substances we cannot do without—light and oxygen! Free radicals, components of oxygen metabolism, damage or inactivate components of cell membranes. Light can loosen the bonds of molecules in skin cells, making them even more prone to free radical damage.

The body is naturally equipped to reduce harmful levels of oxidizing agents, but the job can only be done well with all the right tools, including good nutrtion and nutritional supplements. Some of the best known antioxidant supplements are the vitamins A, C and E.

Once again, the spotlight is falling on vitamin C. Trials, such as one at Duke University on a vitamin C cream, will test how well antioxidant substances are absorbed and their effectiveness. As an antioxidant, it is thought that vitamin C may help guard against wrinkling, declining collagen synthesis, and skin cancers. The theory is that antioxidants help prevent the breakdown of cell membranes. It's believed that a vitamin C skin application could boost the production of skin-firming collagen by special cells called fibroblasts.

Examples of other members of the cooperative antioxidant group are natural plant pigments known as carotenes. The amount of carotene in tissue is considered the most significant factor in determining life span in mammals, including humans! Keeping up carotenes works to boost immune functions active in the skin.

Flavonoids, the major coloring agents in plants, are antioxidants supplied by a green and fruit-filled diet. These compounds are unusual in their activity against a wide range of free radicals and oxidants. In skin and elsewhere flavonoid action works against cancer and is anti-inflammatory, keeping its stress load down and appearance up.

Moisturizers enhanced with antioxidants, although not proven, are probably worth trying. An antioxidant-rich diet, however, seems a very worthwhile measure to keep your skin looking young. To boost your dietary intake of antioxidants try the following supplements:

- Beta-carotene—15,000 IU daily.
- Vitamin C with flavonoids—1000–2000 mg daily.
- Vitamin E (dry form)—400 mg daily.
- Grapeseed extract—150-300 mg daily as a rich source of PCOs.
- Selenium—200 mcg daily.

Smoking and Wrinkling

A report in the *Annals of Internal Medicine* found that smoking greatly increased the chance of facial wrinkling. Obvious examples are the stark lines produced by puckering the lips to draw on a cigarette. Smoking is thought to cause wrinkling in two ways. First, by damaging collagen and elastin, proteins in skin which keep it supple and firm; second, by producing changes in the tiny blood vessels of the face. Stopping smoking could well lead to some reversal of these effects. Yet another reason to add to the long list of reasons for smokers to quit!

Aging, Immunity and Skin

In healthy people, the cells' ability to repair themselves declines at a constant rate of about one percent per year from age 20 to 60, an underlying factor in the tendency for skin cancer to develop in middle age. Fresh skin cells in a healthy 30-year-old typically take about 24 days to move to the outermost layer of skin. By the age of 60, this short journey usually takes twice as long! This means skin is more vulnerable to environmental damage for double the time, with the worst culprit being the sun. Sun protection from early on in life has potentially huge immunity payoffs in old age, since UV rays have been shown to damage the immune system. It's never too late, however, to take protective measures.

Super Skin Secrets of Fruit, Wine, Milk, and Honey

Cleopatra bathing in asses' milk really wasn't such a silly idea. The same goes for rubbing wrinkly elbows with half a lemon. This is because certain plant and dairy food acids, such as honey and molasses, lactic acid in sour milk, salicylic and citric acids from fruits, tartaric acid in wine, grapes and other fruits, and malic acid in apples, promote new cell growth. Known as hydroxy acids (HAs), these substances also cause shedding of dead cells.

Research using sophisticated measuring techniques on the effects of hydroxy acids on skin is now widespread. In one study the researchers had 20 subjects applying a mixture of HAs twice daily over 20 weeks. A control group of 15 people applied the same mixture, but adjusted to neutral rather than acidic. In the unadjusted HA group, a 33 percent increase in cell renewal rates, a 35 percent increase in skin firmness, and a 44 percent improvement in smoothness were seen. Further work shows that HAs seem to achieve most of their moisturizing effect in just two weeks, and their cell renewal and firmness effects in ten to 12 weeks. A very promising result was that improvement in wrinkles and thickness was still increasing at 26 weeks.

The best known HAs are AHAs (alpha-hydroxy acids), but research indicates that all types appear to produce benefits. Hydroxy acids seem to work by naturally increasing the acidity of the skin long enough to loosen cells in the outer layer, stimulating shedding and new cell growth. At a deeper layer, the changed skin acidity may affect enzymes associated with the production of new cells and the skin's inflammatory response. In general, the researchers concluded that HAs do seem to be valuable aids in long-term skin rejuvenation.

For all the benefits, use an HA product with a pH between 3 and 4.5. There have been reports that reddening and cysts can result from HA application in some people. This is thought to be caused by the acidity and may be avoided by using natural sources such as yogurt and honey. The research shows such natural HAs seem to be combined with soothing agents which can even reverse skin irritation. Try some of the recipes in "Soaps, Oils and Lotions for Beautiful Skin" to experience the benefits of HAs.

CHAPTER 5

Nutrition For Beautiful Skin

FOODS FOR BEAUTIFUL SKIN

Fresh fruits, vegetables and whole grains are definitely indicated to keep skin looking beautiful. They are an excellent source of nutrients, including the antioxidant carotenes, and also vitamin C, which is essential for the manufacture of collagen. The following foods in particular will help to ensure a regular supply of skin-enriching substances:

- Cauliflower, lentils, peanut butter, and soybeans—for a supply of biotin, a B-complex vitamin. A deficiency can lead to dry skin and scaliness around the mouth and nose.
- Molasses, tofu, broccoli and sesame seeds—rich sources of calcium; an enzyme in skin is calcium-sensitive, making it an aid in controlling cell functions.
- Whole-grain breads and cereals, beans, shellfish and dark, leafy vegetables—these supply a host of useful substances, including copper, which boosts red blood cells and enhances skin tone and texture because it aids the synthesis of both elastin and collagen in skin.
- Brazil nuts, organ meats and whole grains—particularly for selenium which works well with vitamin E. Selenium binds with an antioxidant enzyme and so helps prevent free radical damage. Brazil

nuts are grown in selenium-rich soil, and one daily should provide enough of this mineral. Soil conditions make other foods a more variable source.

- Salmon, sardines, mackerel, herring and tuna—two to three servings per week of these fish, especially baked or poached, will help you keep up a supply of omega-3 fatty acids. These are essential for healthy cell function.
- Walnuts and canola oil—these are vegetarian sources of healthy fatty acids, but are only about one-fifth as potent as marine omega-3s.
- Berries (especially bilberries, blueberries and elderberries)—an excellent source of the antioxidant PCOs which help maintain the structure of collagen.

SUPPLEMENTS FOR BEAUTIFUL SKIN

Beautiful skin is healthy skin. A smooth, firm, glowing complexion is the result of millions of cells working efficiently and in balance with each other thanks to a continuing supply of water and valuable nutrients. Skin is repaired through constant renewal of its cells and the regulation of their functions.

In a polluted world with a thinning atmosphere, a healthy, whole-food diet, exercise, sunscreen, and sensible use of supplements are essential for beautiful skin. Be persistent. Results can take up to 12 weeks to show. Below are generally recommended supplements all involved in the production or healing of skin cells:

- Beta-carotene—10,000 IU daily. Beta-carotene is converted by the body into vitamin A, an antioxidant which boosts the immune system and is well known for relieving skin problems.
- Vitamin B-complex—100 mg daily will keep you

topped up with several important substances: Biotin, to guard against dryness; pyridoxine, to help fight blackheads and whiteheads and protect against cancer; niacin, for maintenance of general skin health indirectly through its role in the healthy metabolism of fats, carbohydrates and proteins; riboflavin, which is needed more if you are exercising—a deficiency will lead to dry, cracked lips.

- Vitamin C (with bioflavonoids)—2,000 mg daily to promote collagen production.
- Vitamin E (dry form)—400 mg daily of this anti-oxidant anti-aging vitamin which works with vitamin C.
- Zinc—15 mg daily as an immune booster involved in the repair of skin tissue.
- Black currant oil—1,000 to 2,000 mg daily as a supply of essential fatty acids.
- Grapeseed extract—150 to 300 mg daily of this rich source of antioxidant PCOs.
- Glucosamine—an amino sugar naturally occurring in the body, that keeps cartilage strong and flexible, and is a foundational building block and strengthener in the tissue between cells in the skin and mucous membranes. Take it in the form of glucosamine sulfate, n-acetyl glucosamine or Glucosamine/Mucopolysaccharide Complex.
- Herbal infusions—red clover, dandelion and burdock root are particularly helpful. Red clover is often used to treat skin disorders, and it is rich in saponins which boost the immune system and protect against cancer. Dandelion is a useful source of the skin vitamin A and other vitamins, minerals, and chemicals which cleanse skin tissue. Burdock, another tissue cleanser, is antimicrobial and frequently used to relieve conditions like acne.

CHAPTER 6

Natural Preparations for Beautiful Skin

Moisturizing and nutrients are essential for boosting and maintaining the many important functions of skin, with the bonus that skin working well looks great, too. Homemade skin preparations will often be as effective as, if not more so than, expensive commercial preparations. If you do prefer the convenience of ready-made products, seek out those with whole and natural rather than synthetic or derived ingredients. This will provide you with nature's own ingenious safeguards. Fruit acids, for example, may well produce the same beneficial effects as vitamin A-derived treatments such as Tretinoin and Retin-A without the side effects. Recent research suggests that long-term regular use of natural, effective products brings continuing benefits. Be patient! Allow at least two weeks for benefits to begin to show.

QUICK AND EASY LOTIONS

Try the following recipes for skin care lotions, building your favorite into your daily routine, unless your skin does prove sensitive to some of the more acidic ingredients:

- Aloe—this wonderful natural substance is found in many commercial products, but is best scooped fresh from inside the aloe leaf. Full of healing chemicals, aloe is very cooling and soothing. Mix aloe with a little vitamin E if you find it drying.

- Brewer's yeast—this has been found to increase collagen production when mixed with a little water, wheat germ oil or yogurt and patted gently onto the skin. Rinse off once dry.
- Honey—a daily coating allowed to dry for five minutes before rinsing off is a very effective skin cell regenerator.
- Mayonnaise and egg yolk—mix the yolk with ¼ cup of mayonnaise and apply several times a day as an anti-wrinkle lotion.
- White grapes—cut in half and apply gently to the skin around eyes and mouth. A handful of grapes straight from the blender makes a refreshing and toning mask to leave on for twenty minutes before rinsing off. The French have long used champagne to tighten loose skin!

SOAPS AND OILS

Plant extracts, oils and essential oils have been used for hundreds of years for cleansing and healing skin. Follow tradition and make your own concoctions or buy products made with natural, soothing or stimulating ingredients like these:

- Fruit kernel, jojoba, castor and olive oil, are all good for moisture loss. Shake two cups of one oil or a half a cup of all together with a drop or two of a natural (not synthetic) essential oil such as . . .
- Tea tree oil—a powerful antiseptic, healing agent.
- Comfrey oil—to encourage new cell growth and healing.

- Eucalyptus oil—an antiseptic pain reliever that clears the head and stimulates blood flow.
- Lavender oil—used for centuries for its antibacterial, healing and soothing powers.

Add your oil mixture to a warm bath and enjoy not more than a ten-minute soak. Any longer creates dehydration. Alternatively, use one oil at a time to savor its individual properties. Herbal rinses make wonderful facial cleansers. Look for them as ingredients of natural commercial preparations. Use infusions of herbs like those above or try the following:

- Lemon balm (melissa)—used down the ages as a spirit lifter, this herb has antihistamine and antibacterial actions useful against conditions like acne and eczema.
- Chamomile—another antiseptic, very soothing to skin.
- Sage—used by Native Americans as a cleanser and remedy with bear grease for skin sores! Sage is antibacterial and antioxidant.

Whether or not you have a skin condition, it's wise to select products with stimulating or healing agents that naturally tone and condition the skin. Take the trouble to learn what nature has to offer and in just a short time your skin will show the benefits in a firm, smooth and glowing appearance.

PART II:
Beautiful, Healthy Hair and Nails

CHAPTER 7

Healthy Hair and Nail Nutrients

Healthy hair and nails are an outer reflection of inner health. That special shine and vibrancy of healthy hair, and well-groomed fingernails and toenails, send a message to the world about your well-being. When you're sick, malnourished, under stress, or as you age, your hair and nails can become dull and brittle. What's going on? Your hair and nails are made of protein and minerals, and need special nutrients just as much as the rest of you does. If your body is nutritionally deficient, you can bet your hair and nails are too, and may even serve as a warning that something is wrong. When your digestion isn't working or your hormones are out of balance, it will also show up on your head and hands.

In this chapter I will explain how hair and nails work, and introduce you to the nutritional building blocks of hair and nails.

Hair and nails are more than mere decoration. Hair protects the skull by cushioning it, protects the scalp from the sun and wind, and hairs on our eyelashes, and in our nose and ears filter out dust and dirt particles. Our fingernails also serve a purpose. At one time they were probably used as weapons and tools, but they also serve to protect the tips of our fingers and give them extra strength. When we use our hands to grasp something, or when we walk and run, our finger- and toenails provide stability.

THE INNER WORKINGS OF HAIR

Each individual head hair has a lifespan of between two and six years, with three cycles. The first is a "growing" cycle, the second is a "resting" cycle which lasts for only a few weeks, and the third is the "falling" cycle when it dies and falls out, to be replaced by a new hair. Most head hair grows about half an inch per month, faster in the summer, and we normally shed 50-100 hairs a day.

Hair grows from follicles, or sacs beneath the skin that contain the root of the hair, much as a pot contains a plant. The average number of hairs on a head is 100,000. The root of the hair is surrounded by a bulb that feeds it with the tough fibrous protein, keratin. Each tiny hair follicle has its own blood supply, making good circulation a key to healthy hair! The size of the opening in the follicle determines the thickness of the hair. Relative to its circumference, hair is very strong—stronger than a copper wire of the same thickness.

Hair color is genetically determined, and caused by a pigment called melanin found in the follicle. The basic colors are red, yellow, brown and black, but most hair is a combination of these colors. It is the decline of melanin production that causes hair to lose its color, turning gray, which is its original color mixed with white, or white, which is a complete absence of melanin.

Attached to each follicle are tiny muscles called erector pili, which contract when you're cold or scared. This is what makes animals' hair stand on end, creating a layer of warm air between the erect hairs. Though we no longer have hair covering our bodies as fur, we still have erector pili muscles, which can be seen in action when we have goose bumps.

Just above the bulb and below the skin are sebaceous glands, which produce an oily substance called sebum which lubricates and protects the hair.

The shaft of hair is made of three layers: the center core or medulla, the thicker middle layer, called the cortex, and the tough outer layer, the cuticle. Hair is straight, curly or wavy depending on the shape of the hair shaft. Straight hair has a round shaft, curly hair has an kidney shape and wavy hair has a slightly curved shaft.

THE INNER WORKINGS OF NAILS

Fingernails and toenails grow from near the bone about a quarter of an inch past the base of the nail. This is called the nail root. Forming a protective barrier between the nail and the skin is a flap of tissue called the cuticle. Improper trimming of the cuticle can allow bacteria and fungi to enter the sensitive tissue under the nail, causing unsightly nails and painful infections.

Under the nails is the nail bed, which is rich with blood vessels and very sensitive. The pink color of the nails is caused by blood vessels close to the surface.

The nails are made of a tough protein with a high sulphur content called keratin, produced by the cells under the nail. Fingernails grow about an eighth of an inch per month, and toenails grow about a sixteenth of an inch per month. As with hair, fingernails grow more quickly during the warm summer months.

At one time it was said that eating gelatin would create strong nails, but this is a myth. Both hair and nails are composed primarily of protein, and gelatin is far from being a complete protein. It is also a myth that calcium will build stronger nails—the amount of calcium in nails is minimal. There is very little you can do to create hard nails from the outside. Good nutrition and genetics will determine your nail strength. If you have brittle or soft nails, it is especially important to make sure you're getting all of the B vitamins in abundance, not only from eating enough high quality protein, but also in a supplement.

NUTRITION FOR HEALTHY HAIR AND NAILS

Protein

Hair and nails are 98 percent protein, so you can probably guess what your key nutrient is when it comes to healthy hair and nails. Although protein is the basic building block of hair and nails, too much will do more harm than good. And since hair loss is associated with a high-fat diet, you need to get the majority of your protein from low-fat sources such as fish, poultry and legumes such as soy.

For most of us in Western cultures, getting enough protein is not an issue—in fact most of us get too much protein. Too much protein can also cause unhealthy hair by making the body too acidic. The kidneys need to buffer acidic substances with calcium before they are excreted in the urine. Too much protein will cause a calcium deficiency, which will deplete it from your hair and nails.

Vitamin A

Vitamin A is a key vitamin for healthy skin and hair and nails. One of the signs of vitamin A deficiency or excess is hair loss and soft or brittle nails. If you're eating your five servings of fruits and vegetables a day, you'll be getting lots of vitamin A in yellow and orange vegetables and fruits, and dark green leafy vegetables such as kale and broccoli. Other sources of vitamin A are liver, egg yolks, milk and butter. You should be taking 10,000 to 15,000 IU of beta-carotene in your daily vitamins, which the body will convert to vitamin A as needed.

Vitamin E

Vitamin E is the other key vitamin for healthy hair and nails. I recommend that everyone take 400 IU of vitamin E daily. Food sources of vitamin E are unrefined, extra virgin olive oil, whole grains, avocado, and nuts.

A Healthy Thyroid Gland

A healthy thyroid gland is essential for healthy hair and nails. Dull, lifeless hair and fragile nails can be caused by a thyroid deficiency. Iodine is important for proper thyroid metabolism. It's found naturally in fish, and is added to most table salt. The Chinese get their iodine by adding a variety of dried seaweed to their foods. Try adding some wakame, hijiki or arame seaweed to miso soup, and you'll be getting your iodine and many other minerals, along with your low-fat protein! Excessive estrogen, especially relative to low progesterone, can block thyroid action. If your hair has turned lifeless since menopause, try some natural progesterone cream.

Iron

Iron is an important mineral in hair and nail health, but iron deficiencies in adults are actually quite rare, and recent research indicates that too much iron can set up damaging oxidation reactions in the body. I recommend you get small amounts of iron in your multivitamin. Otherwise, don't be concerned with it unless you are anemic.

Cysteine

Cysteine is an amino acid (one of the building blocks of protein) found in large amounts in the hair and nails. Eggs, meat and dairy products are good sources of cysteine, but since they are high in fat, you can also take cysteine capsules, up to 1,000 mg daily, on an empty stomach. (If you are diabetic or allergic to monosodium glutamate, do not take cysteine.)

The B Vitamins

All of the B vitamins are important to healthy hair and nails. Biotin is especially important. This member of the B-complex family is actually added to many shampoos. However, it will do you more good on the inside than the outside. Although a biotin deficiency is rare, it can cause hair loss, dry skin and fragile nails. Biotin can be depleted by low calorie weight-loss diets, oral antibiotics and a steady diet of raw egg whites. Eating foods high in biotin such as nuts, whole grains, organ meats, such as liver, and vegetables, can reverse hair loss caused by a biotin deficiency.

Selenium

This important mineral is both a potent antioxidant and acts as an enzyme for many important bodily functions. Healthy hair, skin and nails are all dependent on sufficient selenium in the diet. You should be getting 100–200 mcg of selenium daily.

Silica/Silicon

After oxygen, silicon is the most abundant element in the earth's crust. It is also abundant in the human body and plays an important part in maintaining the architecture of hair, skin and nails. Collagen, the "glue" that holds our tissues together, contains a large proportion of silicon. In our blood, silicon is found in the same concentration as it is found in sea water. Some researchers speculate that a decline in silicon levels in the body contributes significantly to the aging process.

In laboratory studies, deficiencies of silicon in rodents induced cartilage and bone disease and damage. Furthermore, when the diets of rats with broken bones were supplemented with silicon, they healed faster than those not receiving silicon. Silicon is present in abundance in whole foods, such as whole grains, and fresh fruits and vegetables.

A form of silicon, called silica, is used as a dietary supplement for healthier hair, skin and nails. The horsetail plant is used as a source of vegetable silica, and silica gel is derived from quartz crystals.

If you have brittle nails and hair loss, you may have a silicon deficiency. Try taking silica supplements in the form of horsetail or silica gel for three or four months. You can find it at your health food store.

Glucosamine

Glucosamine is an amino sugar made in the body from glucose and amino acids. Glucosamine keeps cartilage strong and flexible, and is a foundational building block and strengthener in the tissue between cells in the skin and mucous membranes. A deficiency of glucosamine can lead to weakness in these tissues. Take it in the form of glucosamine sulfate, n-acetyl glucosamine or Glucosamine/Mucopolysaccharide Complex, 1000 mg daily in divided doses.

CHAPTER 8

What You Can Do to Prevent Hair Loss

Both men and women hate to lose the hair on their head, but men suffer from baldness more than women do. Ever since Delilah relieved Sampson of his hair, and thus his manliness, Western cultures have equated men's hair with youth and virility. Studies exploring cultural attitudes about balding show that men with hair loss are seen as more passive, less likely to be successful and less likable. According to one study, the only characteristic not perceived as diminished by baldness is intelligence.

A single scalp hair has a two- to six-year growth cycle. What happens on your head during that cycle depends on your diet, your health, your genes and your hormone balance. Most people lose 50 to 150 hairs a day. More than this, and you may find yourself with thinner hair. If you notice when you shower that you're losing more hair than usual, take note of your health.

Some 20 to 30 million men in America alone are bald or balding. The most common type of hair loss in men is known as *androgenetic alopecia,* or male pattern baldness (MPB). Some 95 percent of baldness is MPB, and it is caused by male hormones. It is thought that changes in testosterone cause the hair follicles on the head to begin producing the thin "peach fuzz" or *vellus* hair that covers much of the body, instead of the heavier, darker *terminal* hairs normally produced on the head. Balding men may lose 150 to 300 hairs daily.

Women may lose hair during pregnancy and after menopause, when androgens, or hormones that confer male attributes, become more dominant than estrogen and progesterone. While men go bald, women's hair tends to thin out over the entire scalp.

The only substance approved by the FDA for treating baldness is minoxidil (Rogaine). This drug was originally sold as a hypertensive (lowers blood pressure), but people who took it—men and women—began reporting excessive hair growth all over the body. Its maker, Upjohn, quickly put it into clinical trials as a medication to restore hair growth. Although minoxidil has since been approved by the FDA for this use, in truth minoxidil doesn't work very well, and never completely restores hair. Men whose hair is thinning can get a small benefit from the drug as long as they take it, but when they stop, the hair will just fall out again. And meanwhile, minoxidil is a powerful hypertensive with many side effects of its own and is very expensive.

POSSIBLE CAUSES OF HAIR LOSS

Aging
Genetic predisposition
Prescription drugs (birth control pills, anticoagulants, chemotherapy)
Fungal infections
Radiation
Immune disorders
Diabetes
Iron deficiency
Vitamin C deficiency
Vitamin B deficiency

Zinc deficiency
Excess vitamin A
Progesterone deficiency in women
Hypothyroidism (low thyroid)
Poor diet (especially lack of protein)
Pregnancy (usually grows back within three months
after delivery)
Silica/silicon deficiency

Hair Loss and Illness

Hair loss can be caused by many types of illness, including allergies and particularly celiac disease (intol-
erance for wheat gluten), diabetes, and autoimmune
diseases such as lupus. Hair loss can also be associated
with a high-fat, high-sugar diet. In Chinese medicine,
too much "sweet" consumption is associated with hair
loss. Hair loss can also be caused by skin disorders
such as eczema and psoriasis.

Hair Loss and Aging

If you're a woman of menopausal age and your hair
is starting to fall out, you may be deficient in the
hormone progesterone. Many women are familiar with
the hair loss immediately following pregnancy, which
is caused by a dramatic drop in progesterone production. Using some natural progesterone cream will
quickly restore hair growth for most women.

Hypothyroidism, or low thyroid, especially in
women, can cause hair loss. If you have other symptoms of hypothyroidism, such as cold hands and feet,
fatigue and unexplained weight gain, see your doctor
for a thyroid test.

Vitamins and Herbs For Preventing Hair Loss

Since hair follicles are fed by blood vessels, good circulation is also a key to good hair. There are many vita-

mins and herbs that help circulation. Ginkgo biloba, an herb that improves circulation to the extremities, may just improve your outer brain beauty as well as your inner brain power! Coenzyme Q10 is an important substance for senior citizens whose circulation isn't as good as it once was. Many people who take coenzyme Q10 every day report that their hair is thicker and shinier. Niacin improves circulation to the scalp, and there is some anecdotal evidence that it slows the process of hair loss in men.

Vitamin E and vitamin C both improve circulation, and the bioflavonoids strengthen capillaries which feed the scalp. Vitamin E supplementation can also reduce testosterone levels in women, which may halt the process of hair loss. A zinc deficiency can compromise the immune system and contribute to hair loss. Be sure you're taking at least 15 mg of zinc daily. Deficiencies of vitamin A and vitamin C can also contribute to hair loss. Be sure you're taking 15,000 IU daily of beta-carotene to get your vitamin A, and be sure to take at least 1,000 mg daily of vitamin C.

CHAPTER 9

Keeping Your Hair and Nails Healthy

Hair and nails are often subjected to what I call "hair abuse" and "nail abuse." This abuse is often dictated by the tyranny of fashion which drives us to dye our hair, style it with spray and gels, perm it, blow dry it and expose it to sun and wind. It also drives women to put strange colors on their nails and subject them to drying polishes and polish removers. The same things that dry out the skin will dry out the hair and nails: low humidity, constant exposure to water and soap from doing dishes and other housecleaning chores, sun, wind, and chlorine.

We've all noticed that our hair is less than shiny and lustrous after we've been swimming in a chlorinated pool. Sun, wind and salt water also take their toll on hair. How can you have your fun in the sun and have healthy hair too? Like all good answers, this is a simple one: wear a bathing cap in the ocean or pool, and a hat in the sun. If you're going to be in the wind, either wear a hat, or if your hair is long, pull it back in a ponytail or braid. If you don't want to wear a bathing cap, be sure to shower as quickly as possible after coming out of a pool or the ocean. Even just taking a shower, your hair picks up chlorine. I always recommend that if you have chlorinated water you use a shower filter that filters out chlorine, a poison which is absorbed in large amounts through the skin, especially when the pores are enlarged under the influence of warm water.

GRAYING HAIR

Graying hair is a natural part of the aging process for most of us, but one which we tend to resist mightily, as the booming business in hair colorings will attest. There's essentially nothing you can do to prevent graying hair, but you can avoid premature graying with good nutrition, regular scalp massage, avoiding "hair abuse," and minimizing stress.

A vitamin B12 deficiency can cause graying of hair. A deficiency of vitamin B5, pantothenic acid, can also cause graying of hair. In rodents this graying is reversible when B5 is replaced, but this has never been demonstrated in humans. Nevertheless, if you are experiencing premature graying, I recommend you take an extra B-50 complex supplement.

Premature graying can also be caused by celiac disease, thyroid disease, diabetes, pernicious anemia and other autoimmune diseases.

DRY HAIR

Hair abuse is the primary cause of dry hair, although a lack of essential fatty acids (EFAs) can also contribute. If you're eating plenty of whole grains, nuts, seeds, legumes and fresh fruits and vegetables, you should be getting plenty of EFAs. However, hydrogenated oils can suppress EFAs, and can cause deficiencies—yet another good reason to avoid these synthetic oils like the plague!

Hair is normally covered with an oily substance called sebum, which makes it lustrous and shiny. Harsh shampoos, shampooing too frequently, sun, wind, low humidity and chlorine will all pull moisture out of the hair shaft and strip away the sebum. This causes the outer layer, or cuticle of the hair, to crack, exposing the center and causing it to fray or split, leaving hair dry, frizzy and brittle. Conditioners do not repair split ends. The only cure for split ends is to cut them off.

If you have dry hair, use a high-quality conditioner every time you shampoo. Giving your hair an oil conditioning treatment once or twice a week will help. Use olive oil, jojoba, castor or sweet almond oil. Gently work it into your hair, and then comb it through to make sure it is well-coated. Wrap your hair in a towel and leave the oil on for at least 30 minutes.

DANDRUFF

Dandruff is a common disorder of the scalp which causes the skin to scale and flake off, leaving its embarrassing residue on the shoulders. It causes itching, and the resultant scratching results in further irritation of the skin. Dandruff is caused when the natural process of skin shedding is accelerated, probably from a fungal infection. Dandruff can also be caused by dietary deficiencies, stress and "hair abuse" in the form of too much hair dye, perms, excessive blow drying, and so forth.

A deficiency of vitamin A can cause hair to become dull, brittle and the scalp to become dry and flaky. A vitamin B6 deficiency can also cause dandruff, as can vitamin C deficiency in its extreme form.

If you have dandruff that doesn't itch, you're probably abusing your hair. Try avoiding hair sprays and gels, blow drying, dyes, harsh shampoos, perms and straighteners for six weeks and see what happens. In the meantime, you can try a hair rinse of a few drops of essential oil of rosemary, a few drops of tea tree oil, and half a cup of apple cider vinegar in about two cups of water. Massage into your hair after shampooing, and leave there for two to three minutes. Rinse in cool water and gently pat your hair dry.

You can take 100 mcg of selenium daily to relieve flaking and itching.

You can also look for natural dandruff shampoos containing selenium or tea tree oil, which are antifungals.

SCALP MASSAGE

One of the reasons stress is so damaging to hair is that when we're tense we tend to contract our scalp muscles along with all our other muscles. This in turn contracts the tiny muscles around the hair follicles, causing a reduction in oxygen and other nutrients to the follicle.

Massaging your scalp is a key to healthy hair. It increases the flow of blood and oxygen to the hair follicle, improving hair growth and hair quality. I recommend you spend two to three minutes gently massaging your scalp with the tips of your fingers every morning in the shower. Be sure to massage the scalp rather than the hair, to avoid damaging your hair. It's also wonderful to have someone else massage your scalp for you!

HEALTHY HAIR TIPS

- Wash your hair in warm water and rinse it in cool water.
- Use shampoos with natural ingredients—check your health food store.
- Don't apply shampoos or conditioners directly from the bottle. Pour a small amount into the

palm of your hand, dilute it with a little water, and then apply it.

- You don't need to wash twice with most shampoos. Washing once will protect the healthy oils in your scalp and on your hair.
- Use a large, thick-toothed comb to comb conditioner through your hair.
- Rinse out conditioner thoroughly or your hair will be heavy and oily.
- Dry your hair by wrapping it in a towel and blotting it, rather than rubbing it, pulling it or wringing it.
- When your hair is wet, comb it gently, working from the bottom up.
- Protect your hair from the sun and wind, which will dry it.
- Wear a bathing cap when swimming in chlorinated pools.
- Rinse your hair right away after swimming in the ocean.
- If possible, avoid or go easy on hair dyes (most of them contain coal tar, which is carcinogenic), bleaches and perms. They will all eventually make your hair dull.
- If possible, dry your hair naturally. The constant use of hot combs, heated rollers and blow dryers will make your hair dull.

MAINTAINING HEALTHY NAILS

The condition of your nails can tell you a lot about your health. Yellow nails can indicate respiratory disorders, and white nails can indicate liver problems. White spots may be caused by damage to the nail, or may be a sign of folic acid deficiency or zinc deficiency.

Transverse grooves across the nails can be a sign of thyroid deficiency. They may also appear in people who are recovering from a serious illness such as pneumonia. Lengthwise ridges in the nails can be caused by anemia, applying too much pressure when manicuring your nails, and by biting your fingernails.

Wearing rubber gloves when you wash dishes or do housecleaning will protect your hands and your nails from the drying effects of water, chlorine and soaps.

If your cuticles are dry and cracked, try applying vitamin E oil directly to them. You can either break open a gel capsule, or buy a small bottle of vitamin E oil.

If your nails are growing very slowly, are splitting, brittle or soft, review the nutrients for healthy hair and nails, the Mindell Basic Vitamin and Mineral Program and the Mindell Healthy Hair, Skin and Nails Program.

Nail fungus, most often found in the toenails, can be very difficult to treat. It requires daily attention with an antifungal agent. I recommend you use a natural antifungal agent such as tea tree oil, rubbing it into the nails every night before bed.

THE MINDELL BASIC VITAMIN-MINERAL PROGRAM

Not everyone requires the same vitamins/minerals. Here's a basic program. Ideally you'll take a high-potency multiple vitamin at least twice a day that gives you:

- Beta-carotene, 10-25,000 IU.
- B-complex, 50-75 mg each of B1, B2, B6, PABA, pantothenic acid, biotin, choline, inositol, niacinamide, 1,000 mcg of vitamin B12 and 400 mcg of folic acid.
- Vitamin D, 400 IU.
- Vitamin C complex, 500-1,000 mg (with bioflavonoids)

- Vitamin E, 400 IU.

High-potency multiple mineral mix of:

- Calcium, 600 mg.
- Magnesium, 300 mg.
- Iron, copper, zinc, selenium, chromium, boron, manganese, iodine and potassium.

THE MINDELL HEALTHY HAIR, SKIN AND NAILS PROGRAM

- Follow the Mindell Basic Vitamin Program (see page 75)
- Drink 6-8 glasses of clean water daily.
- Get at least 20 minutes of exercise at least five times a week.
- Eat plenty of whole grains (brown rice, whole-grain wheat, millet and rye), nuts and seeds, all of which contain "healthy" oils which nourish hair, skin and nails as well as vitamins and fiber.
- Eat plenty of fresh organic fruits, vegetables and legumes such as soy which contain the fiber for good digestion and the vitamins, minerals and hundreds of phytonutrients so basic to good nutrition.
- Keep meat and fat consumption low. Eat red meat once a week at most or eliminate it from the diet. Eat chicken or turkey two or three times a week, and be sure it's free-range fowl free of hormones and antibiotics.
- Eat fish at least two times a week, preferably salmon, mackerel, cod and other cold-water fish.
- Eat eggs two to three times a week.
- Get plenty of sleep.
- If you're living a stressful lifestyle, learn a "relax-

ation response" such as meditation, biofeedback, yoga, qi gong, tai chi or positive visualization.

Avoid:

- Avoid hydrogenated oils and processed oils. Emphasize extra-virgin olive oil.
- Avoid sugar and refined carbohydrates such as pastries, cookies, etc.
- Avoid fried foods.
- Avoid junk foods, fast foods, canned foods, frozen dinners and other processed foods which are generally "nutrition free" and loaded with additives, preservatives, dyes, salt, sugar and fat.
- Avoid excess caffeine consumption (more than two cups a day).
- Avoid excess alcohol consumption (more than two drinks a day).

REFERENCES

Bauer, J., et al., "Cytokines, Neuropeptides, and Other Factors in Cutaneous Immune Responses," *Western Journal of Medicine*, Feb. 1994, 160:2:181(3)

Cameron, M. *Lifetime Encyclopedia of Natural Remedies*, Parker Publishing, 1993, pp. 129-33, 156-59, 252-54, 328-31, 397-401.

Carlotti, P., et al., "The Cellular Aging Process and Free Radicals," *Drug & Cosmetic Industry Magazine*, Feb. 1989:144:2:22(3)

Carper, J., *Food Your Miracle Medicine*, Harper Perennial, New York, 1994, pp. 14-16, 240-241.

Davies, S. et al., *Nutritional Medicine*, Avon Books, New York, 1990, pp. 20-21, 72, 269-278

Deakin, L., "Summer Tan? New Evidence—Finally Change Your Mind." *Total Health*, Aug. 1993:15:4:54(2)

Donahue, P., "Relief from Chronic Skin Problems," Dell Publishing, New York, 1992.

"Don't Be Stupid Under the Sun," *USA Today* (Magazine), July 1993:122:2578:6(2)

Fenske, N., "Common Problems of Aging Skin," special issue: "Caring for the Aging Patient," *Patient Care*, April 15, 1989:23:7:225(8)

Ganske, M., "Feed Your Face: Why Your Complexion Needs Vitamins," *Redbook*, May 1995, 185:1:59(3).

Gilchrest, B., "At Last! a Medical Treatment for Skin Aging," *Journal of the American Medical Association*, Jan. 22, 1988:259:4:569(2)

Gorman, C., "Does Sunscreen Save Your Skin?" *Time*, May 24, 1993:141:21:69(1)

Hawk, J., "Ultraviolet A Radiation: Staying Within the Pale," *British Medical Journal*, May 4, 1991:302:6784:1036(2)

Health Letter Associates, *The New Wellness Encyclopedia*, Houghton Mifflin Company, Boston, 1995, pp. 296-7, 549.

Health Letter Associates, *The Wellness Encyclopedia,* University of California, Berkeley, Houghton Mifflin Co., Boston, 1991, pp. 275-99.

Hendler, S., *The Doctors' Vitamin and Mineral Encyclopedia,* Fireside Simon & Schuster Inc. New York, 1991, pp. 63-64, 72, 78-82, 373-374.

Hickey, M., "The Beauty Diet: Foods That Help Improve Appearance," *Ladies' Home Journal,* July 1995:112:7:96(2)

Hunter, C., *Vitamins, What They Are and Why We Need Them,* Thorsons, UK, 1978, pp. 63-72, 90.

"If You Don't Succeed the First Time," *Medical Update,* April 1991, 14:10:4(2).

Johns Hopkins University, "Age Weakens Body's Ability to Fix Sun-Damaged Cells,"*Cancer Weekly,* March 1993:12(2)

Kadunce, D., et al., "Cigarette Smoking: Risk Factor for Premature Wrinkling," *Annals of Internal Medicine,* May 15, 1991:114:10:840(5)

Liberty, M., "The Best Skin Protection Under the Sun," *Better Nutrition for Today's Living,* July 1994:56:7:56(4)

Loughram, J., "Skin Care Basics," *Let's Live,* 55, Jan. 1996.

Mabey, R., et al., *The New Age Herbalist,* Collier Books, Macmillan, New York, 1988, pp. 46, 140-44, 140, 210, 230-33.

Mindell, E., *Earl Mindell's Herb Bible,* Fireside Simon & Schuster, New York, 1992, pp. 38, 43, 60, 83-84, 101, 113-14, 115, 139, 165-6, 221-22, 224.

Mindell, E., *Earl Mindell's Vitamin Bible,* Warner Books, New York, 1991, pp. 31, 41, 53, 52, 55, 60, 62-64, 75, 78, 79, 91, 92, 93, 120, 137, 149-53, 178-80, 212, 214, 216, 221-22, 279-80, 283-85, 288, 318.

Murray, M., et al, *Encyclopedia of Natural Medicine,* Prima Publishing, Cal., 1991, pp. 64, 103-9, 157, 197-203, 296-300, 328, 330, 387, 389, 461, 502-6, 536-40.

Murray, M., *The Healing Power of Herbs,* Prima Publishing, Cal, 1995, pp. 35, 180, 324, 362-3.

"Out, Out, Darned Spot! Reducing Liver Spots & Wrinkles with Tretinoin," *Executive Health's Good Health Report*, June 1992, 28:9:8(1)

Potts R, et al., "Changes with Age in the Moisture Content of Human Skin," *Journal of Investigative Dermatology*, 1984, 82:97-100.

Rafal, E., et al., "Topical Tretinoin (retinoic acid) Treatment for Liver Spots Associated with Photodamage," *New England Journal of Medicine*, Feb. 6, 1992, 326:6:368(7)

Reuben, C., "No More Dry Skin," *Let's Live*, Jan. 1996.

"Save Your Skin," *The Edell Health Letter*, Dec.-Jan. 1990:10:1:7(1)

Scwartz, M., "Skin," *Inner Health Group*, Texas, issue 3310.

Shepherd, S., "Smoothing Skin Wrinkles: What's New Under the Sun?" *Executive Health Report*, April 1990:26:7:2(2)

Simons, A., et al., *Before You Call the Doctor*, Ballantine Books New York, 1992, pp. 149-75.

"Skin Problems Among the Elderly," *Medical Update*, Jan. 1991, 14:7:4(2)

Smith, W., "Hydroxy Acids and Skin Aging," *Cosmetics and Toiletries Magazine*, Sept. 1994:109:9:41(6)

"Tanned Look Grows Old Fast," *The Edell Health Letter*, May 1992:11:5:6(1)

The Dorling Kindersley Visual Encyclopedia, Dorling Kindersley Publishing Inc., New York, 1995, pp. 120.

Thomas, P., "Vitamin C Eyed for Topical Use as Skin Preserver," *Medical World News*, March 1991:32:3:12(2)

University of Texas/Oregon State University "Immune Suppression Caused by Sun Exposure," *NCI Cancer Weekly*, Sept. 4, 1989:4(2)

"Vitamin E Supplementation and Skin Photoprotection," *American Family Physician*, March 1995:51:4:956(1)

Weil, A., *Natural Health, Natural Medicine*, Houghton Mifflin, Boston, 1995, pp. 207, 218, 236, 267, 269.

INDEX